Dedication

This book is dedicated to three beautiful women of color; matriarchs of my family;

Granny, Mommy and Aunt Jerry
You have shaped my positive self-image and cultural awareness. I love you

k

For speaking engagements or Esther's Glow Presentations contact us
At esthersglow@gmail.com

ISBN-13: 978-0-9711021-2-5

Copyright @ 2014 all right reserved.

Library of Congress Cataloging-in-Publication Data

Published by Shepherd Shield Publishing

Graphics and photos by freedigtialphotos.net

Visit us at www.esthersglow.com join our newsletter, look for our upcoming events and share your journey to wellness

Table of Contents

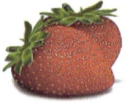

Introduction

<u>**Commentary**</u>

Section I
Why do it!..1

Section II
The Source of our trouble............3

Section III
Seeking Alternatives...................13

<u>**Recipes**</u>

Fast Food................................16

Hearty Healthy.........................31

Sweets for the Sweet.....................................38

INTRODUCTION

In order to maintain proper health and well-being, many nutrients are needed for our body. The Food and Drug Administration (FDA) has formulated their recommendation of a high fiber, well-balanced diet that includes an abundance of vegetables and fruits.

Women of the African and Latin Diaspora have a rich culture and a history that has influenced their eating habits. In addition, socio-economic conditions have also richly impacted their diets. Unfortunately, as a result; high fat, "comfort" foods dominate.

Food has become a source of escape and pleasure, to the detriment of our health and well-being. Before change can occur, there must be a true re-programming of our attitude towards food as a primary source of nutrients.

Many women complain that they want to change their eating habits, however they are limited by finances and time. To add insult to injury, fast-food chains and take-out restaurants have sabotaged our eating routine with easy accessible high sugar and fat content foods.

Do not fret! These recipes can be used for dinner, entertaining, packed lunches or as a mid-day snack. They are low in fat and exclude beef and pork. By utilizing these recipes I have successfully lowered my diagnosed hypertension with moderate exercise. Perhaps after consultation with your physician you may have some of the same wonderful results.   **You will enjoy!**

Who was Esther? She was a Jewish woman who became the Queen of Persia in 457 B.C. Her rise to position was a result of her ability to purify herself and concentrate on her beauty and wellness over many months. Her beauty, courage, wisdom, strength and love for her people culminated in saving the Hebrew Nation from annihilation in the days following Babylonian captivity.

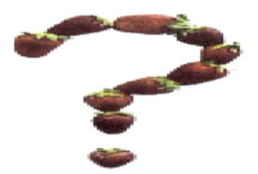

Section I

Why do it!

Section I
Why Do It?
It does not matter what I look like on the outside, GOD looks on the inside....... Why bother?

Many believe that the focus on wellness is vain, not Godly or religious.

On the contrary, the Holy Bible is filled with references to healthy living and wellness. The original sin was centered on "The Forbidden Fruit". The infamous portrait and account of Christ's "Last Supper" and the story of Esther, the inspiration of this book, began with a Feast.

"What:? Know ye not that your body is the temple of the Holy Ghost which is in you, which ye have of God, and ye are not your own? For ye are bought with a price: therefore glorify God in your body, and in your spirit, which are God's" (KJV. 1 Corinthians 6:19-20).

We have a responsibility to take care of our temple; which is our body. We must be conscious of what we put into our body and refrain from eating toxic, and nutrition deficient food.

"Beloved, I wish above all things that thou mayest prosper in health, even as thy soul prospereth." (KJV III John 2)

Why Do It? A 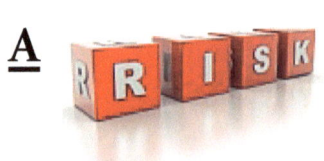 Dangerous Epidemic and Crisis

According to the Center for Disease Control (CDC), 82% of African-American women population are overweight or obese. This statistic can be attributed to unhealthy eating habits and minimal exercise.
It is killing us...

Obesity, high-fat diets, and lack of regular physical activity have been linked to an increase risk for breast cancer recurrence, hypertension and premature death.

The scary thought is that we are passing this death sentence to the next generation, our daughters and sons. There has been an enormous increase in the reports of obesity in our children.

> **Try a little experiment. Stand on any average American city street corner and observe the women who pass by. I guarantee that you will see an overwhelming number of Women of Color who are overweight or obese, compared to their Caucasian or Asian sisters.**

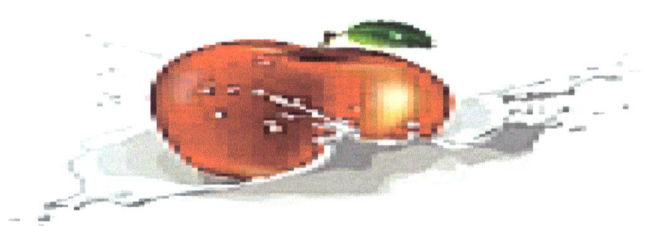

Section II
THE SOURCE OF OUR TROUBLE
Why do we overeat or choose unhealthy foods?

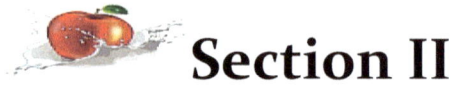 # Section II
THE SOURCE OF OUR TROUBLE
Why do we overeat or choose unhealthy foods?

Now that we know beginning the process is worth it, we must examine the source of our indulgence.

Everywhere you turn, television, books, movies, radio, everyone is talking about wellness. " The Biggest Loser", "Jenny Craig", "Weight Watchers", "Bally's Total Fitness" and print ad magazines with super skinny models; they all bombard us with the same message "look at us, be skinny, be happy, be healthy, you can do it. So what is the problem? Many people continue to be overweight. The source of our trouble stems from the fact that **we may not know what** we should eat or there may be additional factors that influence how much and what type of food we consume.

A. <u>ACCESSIBILITY</u>
Let's face it, the home cooked meal is rare. More Americans are eating fast food due to accessibility and a fast paced and overextended lifestyle. A large proportion of African-Americans, Latin-American, and other people of color eat more fast food over their Caucasian brothers and sisters. Many consider the fast food chains to be a generational phenomenon.

From the seventies to the millennials, children have grown up in the Fast Food world as a part of their daily existence.

> Fast Food restaurants are everywhere. Consider this, in 1968, McDonalds had 1,000 restaurants. Today, there are over 30,000 restaurants and McDonalds is global. Approximately 2,000 new chains open each year.

The Centers for Disease Control and Prevention ranked obesity as the number one health threat for Americans in 2004. It is the second leading cause of preventable death in the United States and results in 400,000 deaths each year. Approximately 60 million American adults are considered obese, with another 127 million overweight.

Excessive calories are another issue with fast food. A regular meal at McDonalds could consist of a Big Mac, large Fry, and a large drink. The calorie count for the described meal tips the scale 1,430 calories in one sitting. Please note, a diet of approximately 2,000 calories is considered healthy for the entire day.

In March of 2009, the American Journal of Public Health, published a study conducted by Brennan Davis, Ph.D. (School of Business and Management, Azusa Pacific University, Azusa, CA) and
Christopher Carpenter, Ph.D. (Paul Merage School of Business, University of California, Irvine) of over 500,000 youths.

The goal was to examine the relationship between fast-food restaurants near schools and obesity amongst middle and high school students. Their findings were stunning.

Their study revealed that students with fast-food restaurants near their schools:
1) consumed fewer servings of fruits and vegetables;
2) consumed more servings of soda; and
3) were more likely to be overweight or obese than youths whose schools were not near fast-food chains

To make matters worse, growing numbers of fast-food chains are staying open later, in some cases 24 hours. Restaurateurs say the purpose for the late hours is due to the "need" of the consumer. It is questionable how they have come to that conclusion
of the consumer.

Unfortunately, people who eat late at night typically do not burn the calories necessary to counteract late consumption. Weight loss will only occur when an individual burns more calories then they consume.

The Wendy's chain is largely credited with this new late night market since it launched extended hours in the year 2000. In 2005, the evolution took a leap forward when about half of McDonald's 13,700 U.S. stores began offering extended hours.

Indulgence

Avoid Falling into the Eve Syndrome

"And when the woman saw the tree was good for food, and that it was pleasant to the eyes, and a tree to be desired to make one wise, she took of the fruit thereof, and did eat, and gave also unto her husband with her; and he did eat. " (KJV Genesis)

Eve made the conscious choice to indulge. Remember, Eve and her husband were authorized by GOD to eat of every other tree in the Garden. The Garden was full of abundance, however Eve perceived it as not enough. Eve sought after what she knew was not permissible. The Bible says that the Serpent did not force Eve to eat, he merely suggested and proposed an alternative way of thinking. Eve acted upon that suggestion and disobeyed GOD.

The average woman of color consumes 1500-2000 calories in one meal at one setting. Did you know that the Food and Drug Administration (FDA) recommends that women intake only 1500-2000 calories per day. It is really simple mathematics.

Ever wonder why athletes are very fit, although they consume high protein and high carb diets? Athletes require high energy and burn the calories in their physical activities. If we want to counter obesity or high body mass, we must find ways to burn more calories than we consume. We must exercise or increase our physical activity.

Does this sound like us, reaching for that extra piece of sweet potato pie, cheeseburger, or cheese cake when we know we should not have it.

After we indulge there is often a feeling of guilt and shame or even depression. Please do not miss this principle; food does not make us overweight, it is our sin/greed that contributes to our overweight or obese condition. We must first repent and confess of our sin of gluttony and then be ready for GOD to sustain us in the transformation of our mind to make healthier choices.

Moderation is key to our success as people of GOD. We should abandon the "Eve syndrome" and embrace "the promise of Esther". The Bible says that Esther was a woman that was "lovely and beautiful": the Hebrew for lovely and beautiful is literally "beautiful in form and lovely to look at". The bible distinctly mentions Esther's twelve month beautification process in preparation for the King. During biblical times oils were widely used for its antiseptic, deodorizing and anti-fungal properties.

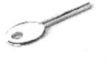 Preparation is Key

The underlying principle we learn from Esther is that we must go through a process of transformation for a beautiful and healthy body. We must eat to satisfy hunger not routinely because something taste good.

Esther was required to spend the first six months before seeing the King preparing herself through a cleansing and purification process.

The story explains that she departed from the "unclean things". The implication is that she became pure in mind, body and spirit before meeting with the king. Esther was revered as a stunning and beautiful woman.

If we adopt the principle of cleansing and preparation we can also obtain the natural glow that is our destiny.

B. *CULTURE*

Many say, just stop eating, start exercising, what is wrong with you? This is easier said that done. First, let us recognize that our bad habits have been developed through years, even centuries of learned behavior and established attitudes towards food.

Historically food has been the one source of comfort for oppressed people. Our food has defined our culture, baked mac n' cheese, sweet potato pie, rice and peas, pork from the "rutta to the tutta", jerk chicken, collard greens, sweet iced tea, country ham, habicheuelas, fried plantains, gumbo, cobblers, fried chicken... should I go on.

These entrees and side dishes are packed with sugar, saturated fat or excess calories. All of them are unhealthy for us if taken on a regular basis.

Ethnic food or soul food is not in itself bad or should not be entirely abandoned. Many of the ingredients of our dishes can be associated directly to resources found in African, Latin-American or Asian countries. For example, the African yam is very similar to the American sweet potato, which is rich in healthy nutrients, such as beta carotene. Rice is a very popular and healthy component of the diet of our West African and Asian brothers and sisters. Another healthy ingredient, collard greens is an excellent source of vitamins and minerals including vitamin A,B,C.

So what went wrong, for those of African-American descent...one word SLAVERY.

Slaves prepared creative dishes to deal with their racial and economic oppression. African-American slaves were not provided with finer cuts of meat by their slave-owners. Many slaves were only offered meats and food that had very little nutritional value. The Slave owners consumed the better part of the farm animals such as milk, butter, and cheese and passed the feet, neck, tails, ears, kidneys, livers and brains to the slaves. (The scraps)

Slaves made the leftover food into gourmet meals by using spices imported from Africa, the Caribbean, and Central and South America. Cornmeal, salt, pork and molasses were stored in bulk by the slave-owners and were frequently distributed to the slaves.

The bulk items and spices added flavor to the bland and bitter leftovers that were given.

Pork fat became the staple for slaves and was used for seasoning vegetables, beans and frying other favorite food such as chicken, fish and white potatoes.

The cultural traditional food had high concentrations of fat, sodium, sugar and starch to season the foods and make it edible. The end result, unfortunately, may have been the seeds for the epidemic that we are currently facing.

People of Color consume large amounts of pork; bacon, pig's feet, ribs, ham, pork rinds, pork chops etc...Pork has been found to be the most widely eaten meat in the world. It accounts for approximately 38% of meat production in the world.

However after these helpful facts, you may want to reduce your pork consumption. Did you know that many cuts of pork have high cholesterol and saturated fat, and excessive consumption can lead to gallstones and obesity.

The pig can be the carrier of various worms such as roundworms, pin worms, hookworms, etc. One of the more dangerous and common worms is the Taenia solium, which is a type of tape worm. Tapeworms may attached themselves to human intestines if transferred by untreated or undercooked meat from pigs or other animals.

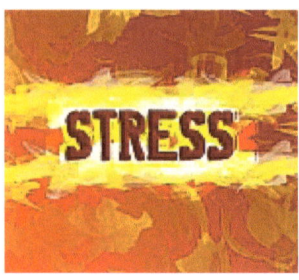

C. *STRESS*

Another contributing factor to obesity among Women of Color is stress. This stress can be directly linked to emotional eating.

What is stress? Stress is our emotional and physical reaction to life. Women of Color deal with many pressures, both financial and emotional. Many are single-parents and have dysfunctional romantic relationships. In addition, racial and gender discrimination may be contributing factors to our emotional eating. You may call it drama, we feel it, stress surrounds our daily living.

Emotional eating has many causes;
   -Biological
Cortisol Cravings: Stress can bring on increased levels of cortisol. Cortisol has been known as "the stress hormone". Cortisol in itself has a beneficial function for the body, however, excessive levels of cortisol brought on by chronic stress can cause many health problems in the body. In fact, high levels of cortisol can create cravings for salty and sweet foods. There is a reason why we call these foods comfort foods.

-Social-Women are social butterfies

We often seek social support under stressful circumstances. Break-ups with boyfriends, parties, movies, salon trips all may frequently include eating sessions with our girlfriends. Crying on your friend's shoulder over a hot plate of barbeque ribs, and a slice of double layered coconut cake is soothing. Going out for a night on the town sharing a plate of fried appetizers and fruity drinks can pack on the calories.

We eat to celebrate and to deal with the pressures of life. Stress may develop as a result of career immobility, marital problems, or financial challenges. We may reach for that slice of cake "comfort food", rather than engage in open and honest communication with our spouse, boss or children. We indulge in food to distract ourselves from feelings of frustration, anger, disappointment and anxiety. This behavior is self-destructive. The result of emotional eating may lead to obesity or hypertension as well as other medical problems.

Stress is a constant factor of our lives, but it is how we mange it that will determine if we survive.

We sedate our minds with food in an attempt to escape the pressures of life. We must develop more constructive and effective ways to manage our stress. Read a book, develop your business, take a dance class, pursue a physical hobby to relieve the stress.

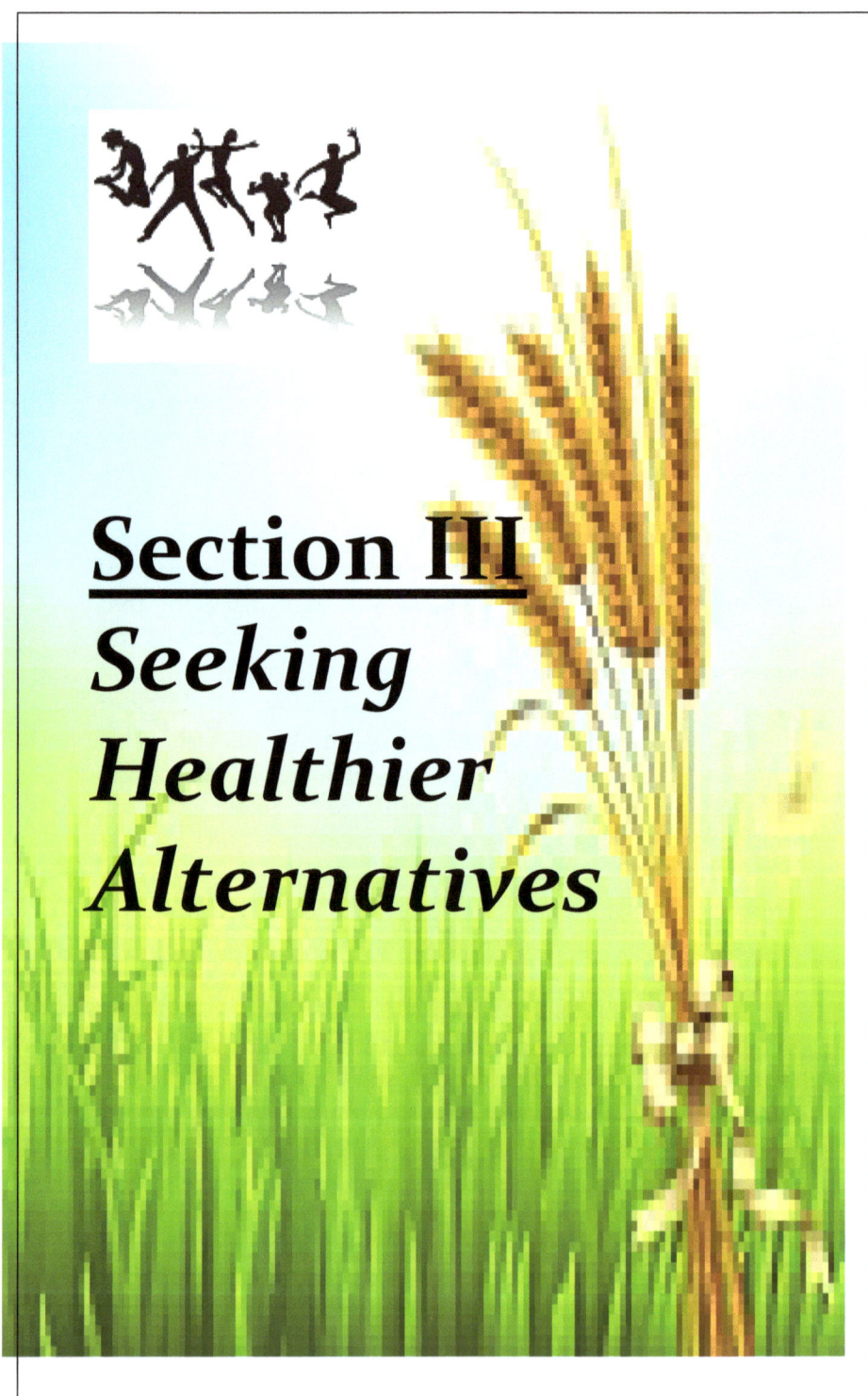

Section III
Seeking Healthier Alternatives

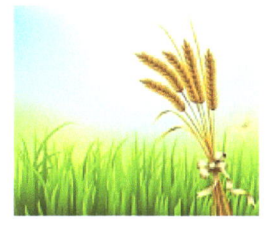

Section III
Seeking Healthier Alternatives

What can we do? The solutions can be found in the following:

Food Choices-
Be more selective in what you decide to consume. Make a conscious decision on the types of foods you will store in your home and eat on the go.

Increase the amount of vegetables you consume. The way to a healthier more energetic you depends upon discipline. Cook your meals and decrease red meat and pork consumption in your diet. We must be conscious of what we put into our body and refrain from eating toxic, or nutrition deficient fast food.

I encourage the reader to use his/her creativity to develop healthier methods of preparation of these beloved cultural foods. Baking at high temperature can be substituted for frying. Steaming and stir frying can be utilized as additional methods.

Make it a point to limit the amount of refined sugars that are called for in recipes. Eliminate sugary drinks like soda from your diet; Soda is packed with high levels of sugar that can be equated to wasted calories.

Use extra virgin olive oil instead of lard, shortening, or butter/margarine recipes. Refrain from using vegetable oils and if necessary substitute it for canola oil.

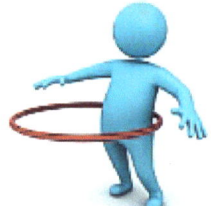

Exercise:

Did you know that physically fit people handle stress more easily than those who are overweight? A regular exercise program such as walking, sports, running, Zumba,etc. is essential to relieving stress and emotional eating. Aerobic exercise helps your body use oxygen more efficiently. Exercise strengthens the heart and lung and relieves tense muscles. Dedicate 15-30 minutes daily to moving your body. Park as far away as you can in a parking lot. Use the stairs instead of the elevator. These little changes over time will make a big difference. Do not be idle.

REST/RELAXATION:
The bible says to meditate on the LORD day and night. Relaxation is a key to managing stress; slow down and enjoy life. We have to make a conscious effort not to conform to the fast paced world that we live.

The bible instructs for us to transform and renew our mind. Do not cram you day with endless chores, set priorities. Plan and designate time to relax in a peaceful environment or space. The space could be as closet, porch or where ever you can find it.

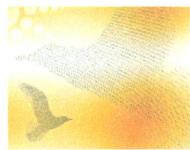 Faith-

We must increase our faith. The Word of GOD, the bible, offers us several stress management strategies. It enables us to develop a positive life style and overall good attitude towards life. GOD knows that it is our nature to become anxious, worried or even doubtful when the pressures of life come our way. GOD love us and has provided us with provision.

> *"Do not let your hearts be troubled. Trust in GOD; trust also in me"*
>
> *"Peace I leave with you; my peace I give you. I do not give to you as the world gives. Do not let your hearts be troubled and do not be afraid." (JOHN 14,1, 27 KJV)*

Find comfort in GOD's word.

FAST FOOD

Recipes

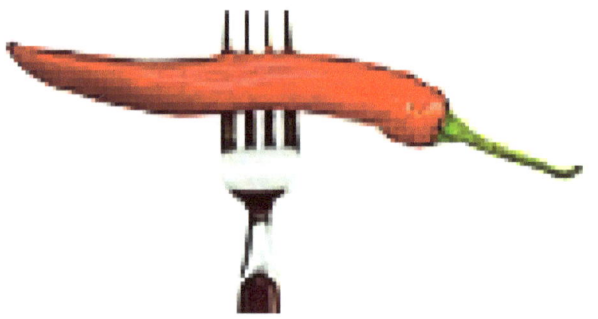

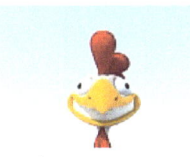

El Poco Loco
Crazy Chicken Wraps

1 ½ cups water
½ teaspoon adobo
3 teaspoons fresh
 Ground black pepper
1 garlic clove minced
½ teaspoon of sazon

3 tablespoons pineapple juice
2 teaspoons juice from a lime
3 whole chicken breast
 (skinned)
1 teaspoon of garlic powder

In a blender or bowl, combine water, adobo, pepper, garlic and sazon. Blend or mix on high for 10 seconds. Gently add the pineapple juice to the mixture and continue to blend for 5 seconds. Marinate the chicken breast for at least an hour. (best overnight)

Grill chicken until no longer pink. Let rest for 5 minutes and slice chicken into five diagonal pieces.

Best served with Loco salso, shredded lettuce and flour or corn tortillas. Use fat free baking spray or grill top to warm tortillas.

Serving size for 2.

Esther's Tip: Invest in an inside grill if you are not able to grill outdoors.

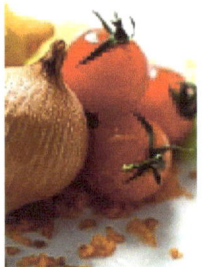

Loco Salsa

2 Med tomatoes   1/2 teaspoon of coarse sea salt
1 fresh jalapeno sliced   1 sprig fresh cilantro
1 med red onion finely chopped
Dash of sugar/or sugar substitute
¼ cup fresh red peppers chopped
¼ cup of green pepper chopped
½ tsp x-virgin olive oil
½ tsp coarse black pepper
Squeeze juice of 1 small lime.
Dash of hot pepper sauce (optional)

Chop the tomatoes, jalepeno together and add onion. Transfer into a bowl. Extract excess liquid.

Add remaining ingredients. Pour salsa into a container and store. Several hours to overnight are best to allow the flavors to develop.

Esther's Tip: Salsa can be delicious w/turkey burgers as a relish or inside a regular or egg-white omelet.

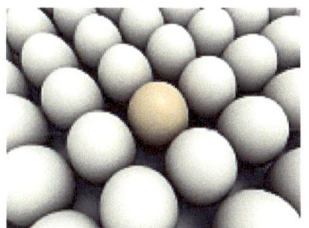

WILD WILD WESTERN OMELET

1 to 2 tbsp. butter
1/2 c. cracked pepper deli turkey, chopped
2 tbsp. Loco *Salsa* (see pg 17)
3 eggs
1 slice of American cheese
2 tbsp. reduced fat milk
1 tbsp Part Skim Cheddar cheese, grated

Melt butter in medium skillet with a little reserved; sauté turkey, peppers and onions until vegetables are tender; set aside. Heat omelet pan or skillet. Add the reserved small amount of butter; coat bottom and sides of pan. Beat eggs, milk, salt and pepper until blended. Pour into omelet pan and cook until eggs are set. Spoon turkey mixture over center of omelet and add American cheese. Fold over, envelope style to hold in filling.

Transfer to serving plate. Top with grated cheese and Serve as breakfast, brunch or a light dinner.

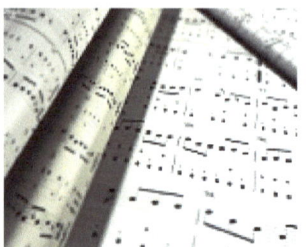

VEGETABLE SYMPHONY
(potatoes, onions, virgin olive oil, kidney beans, spinach, garlic, sea salt, ground pepper)

1 cup of white potatoes
1 can of drained kidney beans
1 cup of fresh chopped spinach
2 cloves of garlic finely chopped
2 medium chopped onions
 1 green onion sliced
¼ cup of extra virgin olive oil

Heat oil, add potatoes and onions until tender. Add garlic, kidney beans and spinach and stir fry for 2-3 minutes add salt and pepper to taste. Drop hint of balsamic vinegar for extra zip.

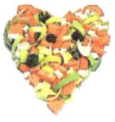

Esther's Tip:
 Good dish when cleansing system

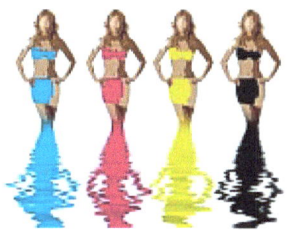

Broccoli Supremes

¼ tsp unsalted butter
1 tsp X-virgin olive oil   ¼ cup orange juice
½ cup shallots, finely chopped
¼ tsp minced fresh ginger   1 tbsp light soy sauce
½ tbsp cornstarch   ½ cup sliced red peppers
1 ½ cup fresh broccoli florets

Add oil and butter to a small sauce pan or skillet on medium-high. Add broccoli and peppers; stir fry for 3 minutes. In a small bowl, combine remaining ingredients. Add broccoli; lower heat and cook until broccoli slightly tender and sauce has thickened, 2-3 minutes.

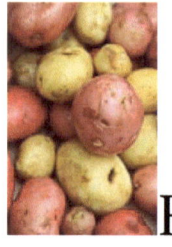

Rusty Roast Potatoes

½ tablespoon coarse salt
4 large all-purpose baking potatoes (cubed)
4 slices of cooked diced turkey bacon
¼ cup of X –Virgin olive oil
1 bunch of chopped scallions or green onions
½ cup of part-skim or low fat cheddar cheese
1 tsp of black pepper (coarse)
1 tbsp of Italian seasonings
½ tsp of garlic powder

In a large pot bring 3 quarts of water to boil. Cut potatoes in cubes. Add potatoes and boil for 6-8 minutes or almost tender. Potatoes should not be completely done. Drain and rinse in cold water.

Toss cooled potatoes in the pepper, salt, Italian seasonings, garlic powder and ½ tbsp olive oil mixture.

In a pan or flat grill heat remaining olive oil over medium heat add turkey bacon, scallions and seasoned potatoes.

Upon potatoes golden brown appearance place in oven safe dish and sprinkle w/cheese on top. Broil for few seconds to melt cheese. Do not burn. Take out of oven and sprinkle chives or extra scallions on top. Delicious!

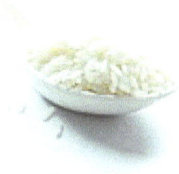

Veggie Fried Rice La Asian

2 tbsp. of X-virgin olive oil
4 scallions, chopped
2 tbsp of chopped fresh garlic
½ cup of shredded carrots
2 cups of left-over white rice
2 tbsp low sodium soy sauce
1 pat of butter

¼ cup Chinese cabbage
(reg will do the job!)
½ cup of green peas
2 eggs beaten
1 tsp of white pepper
1 tbsp. fresh parsley

The key to cooking this dish is prep. Have all veggies and ingredients ready to be put in the pan. Onions.chopped.etc

Heat pan or wok over medium heat; add oil after few seconds or hot, add well drained cabbage, scallions, garlic and ginger. Stir well w/spatula or wooden spoon. Add peas and carrots. Constantly stirring.

Push Veggies to side and make a hole in the center of the veggies to add beaten eggs, butter scramble. Add rice and white pepper to egg mixture, then bring veggies over and add soy sauce.

Esther's Tip: This is delicious as a main course or side dish who needs Chinese take out…

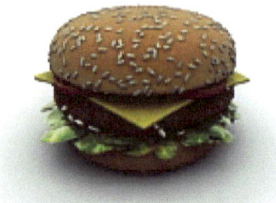

TURKEY BURGERS

(Fast Food the healthy way)

1 pound of ground turkey
1 ½ tbsp of Worcestershire sauce   2 tbsp relish
2 small diced red onions   1 tbsp shallots
½ tbsp X-virgin olive oil   ½ tsp cider vinegar
¼ tsp coarse salt or (substitute)
1 tsp of coarse black pepper

In a large bowl combine the ground turkey, Worcestershire sauce, salt and pepper. Roll portions of meat into a ball and flatten into patties.

Heat olive oil in pan over medium heat and add shallots and onions. Place patties in pan. When one side is cooked flip burgers so the other side and can cook.

Serve or whole grain toasted buns and add your favorite condiments.

Esther's tip: Try making a home made relish in a separate bowl mix red onion, relish, and cider
                              Or
Dress up your burger w/lettuce tomato and loco poco salsa

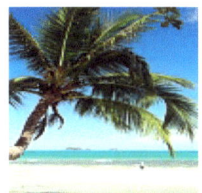

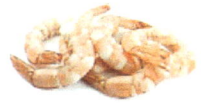

Caribbean *'Mon'* Shrimp

1 lb medium-large deveined shrimp

½ tbsp. of coarse black pepper   1/3 cup water
3 cloves of garlic, chopped   1 small lime
2 tbsp of Jamaican curry powder   ½ cup shallots
1/3 cup of white cooking wine   1 lg white onion
3 tbsp. of X-virgin olive oil   1 tsp of corn starch
¼ cup of chicken stock (no msg, low sodium)
3 potatoes, peeled and sliced

Rinse shrimp, pat dry and season w/black pepper. Heat oil, and add shallots, garlic, curry powder. Then add potatoes and onions and sauté until tender. Stir in chicken stock, white wine and shrimp.

Add cornstarch and little water in a separate cup, mix until smooth. Then slowly add to shrimp pan. Do not overcook shrimp. Shrimp should be opaque. Finish w/juice of lime over the top and garnish.

Esther's Tip: This dish taste fabulous over rice or angel hair pasta.

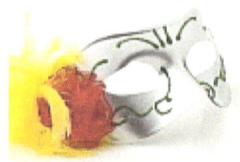

Weesiana-Style Red Beans & Rice

BEANS
One 30 ounce can (low sodium) or two 15 ounce cans small red beans

¼ stick of butter   1 ½ tsp white pepper
¼ tsp paprika   ¼ tsp garlic powder
¼ tsp salt

RICE
1 ½ cup rice   ¼ stick butter
1 cup water   ½ cup chicken stock (low sodium)

Pour beans with their liquid into a large saucepan. Over medium heat add white pepper, garlic powder and salt. When bean begin to boil, use a fork to mask a portion of them against the side of the pan, not all. Stir mix constantly and do not allow to stick.

Prepare the rice, using the butter, chicken stock and water. Boil liquid add rice and cover under low heat until all liquid has evaporated.

Serve by pouring beans over the rice.

Esther's Tip: Delicious when served w/steaming hot buttered cornbread. be modest w/the butter please!

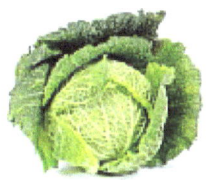

Easy Does it COLESLAW

1 Cabbage head (finely chopped)   1 tsp cider vinegar
¼ cup shredded carrots   ½ tbsp sugar
½ tsp salt   2 tbsp onions
1/8 tsp black pepper   (minced)
2 ½ tbps lemon juice   ½ cup of lowfat miracle whip
½ tsp yellow mustard

Combine cabbage, carrots, onion, sugar, salt, and pepper together in a bowl. Add mustard, miracle whip, vinegar and lemon juice. Lightly toss w/large fork until smooth. Refrigerate in a covered container for minimum of 2 hours before serving for perfection

Esther's Tip: coleslaw can be served as a side or as part of a chopped chicken barbeque sandwich.

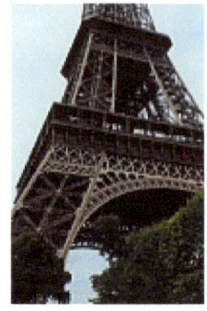

Grilled Chicken
La Dijon Sandwich

2 whole wheat buns   2 green lettuces leafs
2 boneless chicken breast   2 lrg tomatoes slices
1 tsp black pepper (coarse) 1 tbsp honey
2 tbsp Dijon mustard   ½ tbsp low fat miracle whip
½ tbsp. balsamic vinegar (low sodium Salt to taste)

Heat grill or broiler. In a small mixing bowl, add mustard, honey and balsamic vinegar. Set aside ¼ cup of mixture. Marinate chicken breast (boneless/skinless) with the remaining. Before grilling or broiling add the coarse black pepper and salt.

Cook until opaque, completely done. Toast wheat buns. Take the set aside mixture add the miracle whip. Stir and spread over the toasted wheat buns.

Esther's Tip: coleslaw can be served as a side or as part of a chopped chicken barbeque sandwich.

SHRIMP SCAMPI

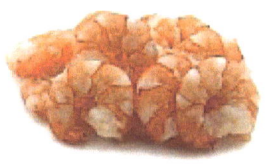

1 lb large shrimp, (peeled & deveined)

1 ½ tsp old bay	½ cup dry white wine
¼ tsp Italian seasoning	1 tbsp minced garlic
1 tbsp X-virgin olive oil	1 pat unsalted butter
½ tbsp cayenne powder	½ tsp black pepper
½ tbsp onion powder	¼ cup lemon juice
1 tsp parsley (chopped)	1 tsp crushed red pepper

Toss uncooked shrimp in a medium bowl w/old bay, Italian seasonings, black and red pepper, onion powder, and cayenne powder.

Place the oil and 1 pat of butter in a large sauté non-stick pan over medium heat. Add shrimp and spread evenly throughout pan. Cook for 2 minutes and turn. Add garlic, then white wine, lemon juice to pan and cook for another 30 seconds, stirring often. Add salt to taste and garnish w/parsley.

Esther's Tip: Serve immediately, over angel hair pasta or herbed rice pilaf.

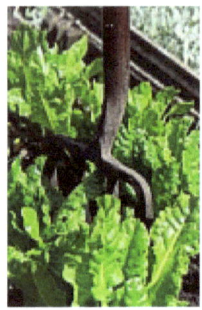

Sautéed Spinach

3 tbsp X-Virgin Olive Oil
2 tsp garlic, chopped
2 tsps shallots, minced
12 ounces of baby fresh spinach
1 tsp of soy sauce (low sodium)
½ tsp of clam juice

In a skillet heat oil over medium heat. Add garlic, then shallots and cook until tender. Approx 1 minute. Add spinach, soy sauce, clam juice for 1 minute or less then remove from heat.

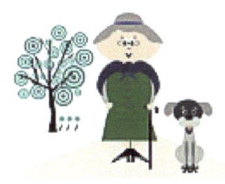

NOT YOUR Granny's GRANOLA

1/2 cup shredded coconut
3 ½ cups old-fashioned rolled oats
1/4 cup unsalted sunflower seeds
1 cup coarsely chopped almonds   1 tbsp. sesame seeds
1/2 teaspoon ground cinnamon
1/4 teaspoon freshly ground nutmeg   1/2 cup honey
1 tablespoons dark brown sugar
½ stick unsalted butter, melted   1/2 cup golden raisins

Heat oven to 350 degrees. Line a baking sheet with parchment, and spread shredded coconut on top. Bake until toasted. Transfer to a wire rack to cool.

Decrease oven temperature to 300 degrees. Line two baking sheets with parchment; set aside. In a large bowl, toss together oats, sunflower seeds, almonds, sesame seeds, cinnamon, and nutmeg. Set aside.

In a small bowl, stir together honey, brown sugar and butter; pour over oat mixture. Stir well. Spread onto sheets. Bake until golden, about 25 minutes. Transfer to a wire rack to cool. Break up granola; sprinkle with raisins and toasted coconut. Store in airtight container

Esther's **Tip:** Oats and other grains are rich in **magnesium** and other minerals and vitamins which help keep cholesterol low. Granola can be a healthy part of a diet rich in natural grains and vegetables.

Hearty Healthy

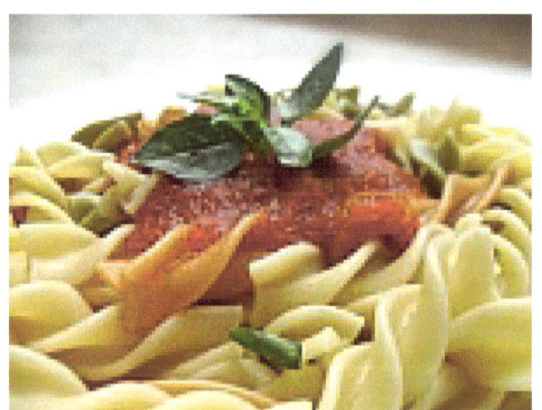

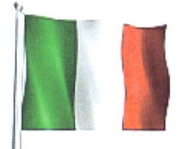

Vega Fun Lasagna

1 bottle of your favorite marinara sauce
1 box lasagna noodles   2 cups of eggplant (cubed)
1 cup of part skim mozzarella cheese (shredded)
1 pkg of ground turkey   ½ cup fresh basil, (finely chopped)
1 pkg Italian hot & sweet turkey sausage
½ cup part skim parmesan cheese
1 clove garlic (minced)   1 (32 oz. can) of tomato puree
½ cups of shallots (finely chopped)
1 red pepper (finely chopped) 1 package of fresh baby spinach
15 oz or 1 tub of part-skim ricotta cheese

Boil noodles separately. Set aside the cubed eggplant and spinach.

Brown sausage and ground turkey in pan. Add garlic, shallots. Combine the rest of the ingredients in a large pot, simmer for a minimum of one hour. In the bottom of a 9' x 13' baking pan, spoon ½ cup of sauce. Cover it with a layer of noodles, follow with a layer of egg plant. Next layer with mozzarella. Build layers w/the remaining noodles, ricotta cheese, spinach, sauce, mozzarella cheese. Top w/ fresh parmesan cheese and fresh basil.

Refrigerate the lasagna until ready to bake. Bake for 45 to 50 minute at 350 degree temperature until bubbly brown. Allow 15 minute to set before cutting and serving.

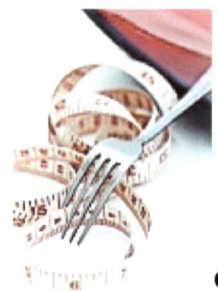

Skinny Ziti

1 box of ziti pasta
3 ½ cup "Quick Marina" (recipe pg 33)
1lb ground turkey
1 tbsp thyme   ½ cup parmesan, freshly grated
1lb Italian Turkey sausage (uncased)
1/2 cup pecorino Romano cheese
½ cup fresh mozzarella (cubed)
1 package of shredded mozzarella cheese

Pinch of crushed red pepper, dash of kosher salt, fresh ground black pepper

Preheat oven to 375 degrees. F. Bring a large pot of water to a boil, add dash of kosher salt. Boil pasta until al dente, tender but still slightly firm. Drain

Brown sausage, ground turkey, with onions and thyme. In a large bowl, toss the cooked pasta with the marina sauce, ¼ cup of the romano and the cubed mozzarella cheese. Season w/black and red pepper to taste and mix until well combined. Transfer the pasta to a fat-free oil sprayed 9'x 13' baking dish. Cover the top of the pasta w/remaining mozzarella and sprinkle w/remaining romano. Bake until lightly browned about 30 minutes.

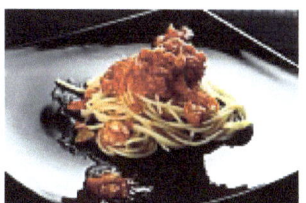

Quick Marinara Sauce

2 tbsp X-virgin oil   1 tsp sugar (or substitute)
¼ med onion (diced)   3 cloves garlic (minced)
3 ½ cups tomato puree   1 roasted red pepper
Sprig of fresh basil   (thinly sliced)
1 ½ tsp kosher salt   dash black pepper (coarse)
½ tsp dried Italian seasonings

Heat the oil in a medium sauce pan over medium heat. Sauté the onion and garlic. Stir until lightly browned about 3 minutes. Add the tomato puree, roasted red pepper and the herbs. Bring to a rapid bowl and lower heat to simmer. Stir in salt to taste and black pepper. Use now or store covered in the refrigerator for up to 3 days or freeze up to 2 months.

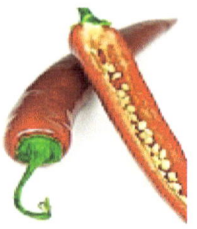

BUF FALO TURKEY WINGS

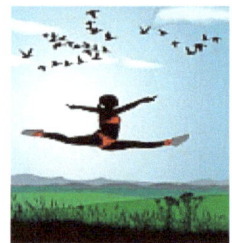

That won't wear you down (fly)

3 pounds turkey wings separated at joints, tips discarded
1 cup Louisiana-style hot sauce
¼ teaspoon cayenne pepper, or to taste
¼ teaspoon ground black pepper, or to taste
1/2 tablespoon Worcestershire sauce
¼ cup melted butter
2 tbsp. thyme   1 green pepper (coarsely chopped)
1 tbsp. seasoning salt   2 tsp of freshly ground pepper
¼ cup of unbleached flour
1 lime

Preheat oven to 325 degrees. Squeeze lime over turkey. Lightly rub wings with butter. Season wings with pepper, seasoning salt, thyme. Toss light coating of flour over wings. and add green pepper. Place in a casserole dish cover and bake for 25 minutes. Uncover and bake until thoroughly done, for a minimum of another 25 minutes. In separate bowl, mix together the hot sauce, melted butter, and cayenne pepper. drizzle sauce to wings and bake additional 15 minutes.

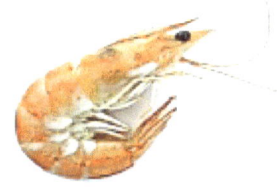

No Guilt Jambalaya

1lb skinless, boneless chicken breast (cubes)
1lb Italian hot turkey sausage, (uncased)
1lb turkey polish sausage
1 lg green pepper, chopped   1 lg onion chopped
1 cup chopped celery   6 cups water
½ tsp dried thyme   1 tsp cayenne pepper
3 cups white rice (uncooked)   2 tsp Cajun season
2 tsp dried oregano   1 cup celery (chopped)
1 (28 oz) can diced tomatoes w/juice
1 cup low sodium chicken broth
1 lb cooked shrimp w/out tails
1 bay leaf

In a slow cooker, mix the chicken, sausage, tomatoes w/juice, onion, green pepper, celery and broth. Season w/oregano, parsley, Cajun seasoning, cayenne pepper and thyme. Cover and cook low for 7 to 8 hours. Stir in shrimp, during the last minute of cooking time. In a large pot, bring the rice and water to a boil. Reduce heat to low and cover. Simmer 20 minutes. Serve the slow cooker mixture over the cooked rice.

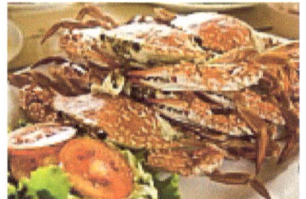

SEAFOOD CHILI

2 tbsp butter
½ cup shallots
½ cup crab meat (lump)
½ tsp white pepper
2 pieces oven fried fish
½ lb med shrimp
1 cup milk (low-fat)
¼ cup mozzarella

3 lg scallops
2 cups of cooked lima beans
1 tsp of old bay
½ tbsp chili powder
¼ cup parsley
1 bay leaf
¼ cup white cheddar
2 cups of cooked rice

Shrimp peel, remove tails, deveined, cut into halves. Scallops cut in quarters. Fish and shallots should be diced.

Heat small pot over med heat. Melt butter, add shrimp, scallops, shallots cook approx 1 minute or until opaque. Stir in Fish and lump crab meat. Add remaining ingredients. Stirring constantly.

Esther's Tip: Great over rice or angel hair pasta

No Guilt Chili

2 lbs ground turkey
(1) 29 oz tomato sauce can
(1) 29 oz can kidney beans
2 tsp cumin powder
1 cup diced onions
½ cup green chili (diced)
½ tsp of sugar
¼ celery (diced)
3 med tomatoes (diced)
3 tbsp. chili powder
1 jalapeno (diced)
1 can tomato paste
2 tbsp. Worcestershire sauce

Season ground turkey w/ worcestershire sauce, black pepper and ¼ cup finely diced onion. Brown turkey in skillet over medium heat until no longer red. Crumble cooked turkey w/fork and place in a large pot. Combine the remaining ingredients over low heat. Stir occasionally for 2-3 hours.

Esther's tip: This savory dish is wonderful w/cornbread on the side.

Sweets for the Sweet

LOOKING SWEET WHILE EATING SWEETS

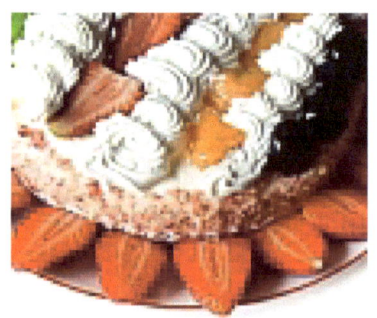

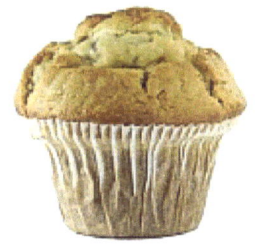

Sweetie Pie Potato Muffins

1 cup 2 or 1% milk
1 egg   + 1 egg white
1 cup cooked sweet potatoes
½ tbsp pure vanilla extract

1 teaspoon cinnamon
1/2 cup honey
1/2 tbsp lemon flavor
3/4 cup golden raisins

1 1/4 cup whole wheat flour
1/4 teaspoon salt
1 1/2 teaspoon baking powder
1/4 teaspoon baking soda

½ cup butter
¼ cup maple syrup

PREPARATION:

Mash sweet potato with lemon and vanilla flavor. Add milk, along with beaten eggs, honey, maple syrup, softened butter and raisins. Mix well.

In a smaller bowl, mix together flour, salt, baking powder and soda. Mix together with the wet ingredients & immediately divide into a butter flavored fat –free oil sprayed muffin pan.

Bake in a preheated oven at 400 <u>degrees</u> for approximately 25 minutes. Let stand for 8 - 10 minutes before removing from pan.

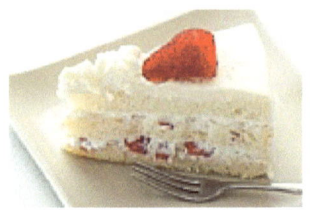

Strawberry Shortcake

1 box of Angel Food Cake Mix
12 oz crushed pineapples
1 cup of fresh strawberries sliced
¼ tsp of pure vanilla extract
1 container fat free whip topping
1 tsp of sugar (or substitute)
1/3 cup of water (room temperature)

Optional add 1/3 cup of coconut to the cake mix and bake

Preheat oven to 350 degrees F. In a mixing bowl add cake mix, vanilla extract and all of the contents of the crushed pineapples. Mix well and pour into two baking oil sprayed round pans. Bake for 45 minutes or as instructed in Cake mix box.

In a small saucepan combine water and granulated sugar. Heat over medium heat until sugar dissolves. Toss strawberries into mixture away from heat.

When cake is thoroughly cooled, use knife to carefully cut the cake horizontally leaving 4 layers. Each layer should receive whipped topping spread over surface topped w/slice strawberries.

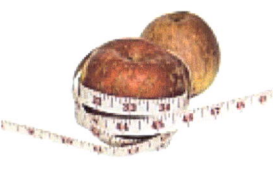

Apple Crumble Crunch

2 green apple (peeled, chopped)   pinch cinnamon
½ cup rolled oats   yogurt
2 graham crackers (crushed)
Brown sugar, honey to taste

Preheat oven to 325 degrees. Mix apple, oats and cinnamon in bowl. In separate bowl mix graham crackers, brown sugar, honey and enough yogurt to make crumbly but not sticky. Spoon mixture over the apple mix and bake for 15 minutes in oil sprayed pan for approx 10 minutes or until apples tender.

~NOTES~

Appendix

A
Apple Crumb pg 40

B
Broccoli Supremes pg 20
Turkey Burger pg 23
Red Beans & Rice pg 25

C
Chicken (El Poco Loco) pg 16
Grilled chicken pg 27
Coleslaw pg 26

Seafood Chili pg 36
No guilt Chili pg 37

G
Granola pg 30

J
Jambalaya pg 35

L
Lasagna pg 31

M
Marinara Sauce pg 33
Sweet Potato Muffins pg 38

P

S
Salsa pg 17
Caribbean Shrimp pg 24
Shrimp scampi pg 28

Spinach pg 29
Strawberry Shortcake pg 39

T
Turkey Wings pg 34

V
Vegetable Symphony pg. 19

Z
Ziti pg. 32

www.ingramcontent.com/pod-product-compliance
Lightning Source LLC
Chambersburg PA
CBHW041753040426
42446CB00001B/18